Fit aı

This Journal Belongs To :

- -

Celebrate your Success!

Reward yourself!

Feel Great Everyday!

90 Day Diet and Fitness Tracker

Daily Exercise, Activity and Food Journal

GOALS/THOUGHTS/PLANS

Celebrate your progress and check off each day of your efforts!

Week 1	1	2	3	4	5	6	7	1
Week 2	8	9	10	11	12	13	14	2
Week 3	15	16	17	18	19	20	21	3
Week 4	22	23	24	25	26	27	28	4
Week 5	29	30	31	32	33	34	35	5
Week 6	36	37	38	39	40	41	42	6
Week 7	43	44	45	46	47	48	49	7
Week 8	50	51	52	53	54	55	56	8
Week 9	57	58	59	60	61	62	63	9
Week 10	64	65	66	67	68	69	70	10
Week 11	71	72	73	74	75	76	77	11
Week 12	78	79	80	81	82	83	84	12
Week 13	85	86	87	88	89	90		13

Measurements:

1. Chest: _____
2. Waist: _____
3. Hips: _____
4. Thigh: _____
5. Calf: _____
6. Arm: _____

Weekly Meal Plan:

Weekly Goals:

_____
_____
_____

How I feel about:

Diet: 😃 😊 😐 ☹️

Exercise: 😃 😊 😐 ☹️

Monday: _____
_____
_____

Tuesday: _____
_____
_____

Wednesday: _____
_____
_____

Thursday: _____
_____
_____

Friday: _____
_____
_____

Saturday: _____
_____
_____

Sunday: _____
_____
_____

Notes: _____
_____
_____

Date: _____ / _____ / _____   Day ⬡ 1

Breakfast: Lunch: Dinner:

_____   _____   _____

_____   _____   _____

_____   _____   _____

_____   _____   _____

Snacks: Cravings / Response:

_____   _____

_____   _____

_____   _____

_____   _____

Calories   Calories   Water Intake:
Consumed: _____   Burned: _____   ⬠ ⬠ ⬠ ⬠ ⬠

Exercise/Workout/Activity: ⬠ ⬠ ⬠ ⬠ ⬠

_____

_____

_____

_____

Weight: _____   Sleep Time: _____   I am Feeling:

                                                      😃 🙂 😐 🙁

How will I make Tommorrow Awesome:

_____

_____

"We are what we repeatedly do.
Excellence, then, is not an act, but a habit."
— Aristotle

Date: ____/ ____/ _____

Day ② 2

Breakfast:

_____

_____

_____

_____

Lunch:

_____

_____

_____

_____

Dinner:

_____

_____

_____

_____

Snacks:

_____

_____

_____

_____

Cravings / Response:

_____

_____

_____

_____

Calories Consumed: _____

Calories Burned: _____

Water Intake:

Exercise/Workout/Activity:

_____

_____

_____

_____

_____

Weight: _____

Sleep Time: _____

I am Feeling:

😃 🙂 😐 🙁

How will I make Tommorrow Awesome:

_____

_____

"Don't count the days, make the days count."
—Muhammad Ali

Date: _____ / _____ / _____   Day ⬡ 3

Breakfast: Lunch: Dinner:
_____   _____   _____
_____   _____   _____
_____   _____   _____
_____   _____   _____

Snacks: Cravings / Response:
_____   _____
_____   _____
_____   _____
_____   _____

Calories   Calories   Water Intake:
Consumed: _____   Burned: _____

Exercise/Workout/Activity:
_____
_____
_____
_____

Weight: _____   Sleep Time: _____   I am Feeling:
                                                     😃 🙂 😐 🙁
How will I make Tommorrow Awesome:
_____
_____

"We cannot start over.
But we can begin now and make a new ending."
—Zig Ziglar

Date: _____ / _____ / _____   Day ⬡ 4

Breakfast: **Lunch:**   **Dinner:**

_____   _____   _____
_____   _____   _____
_____   _____   _____
_____   _____   _____

Snacks: **Cravings / Response:**

_____   _____
_____   _____
_____   _____
_____   _____

Calories   **Calories**   **Water Intake:**
Consumed: _____   **Burned:** _____

Exercise/Workout/Activity:

_____
_____
_____
_____

Weight: _____   **Sleep Time:** _____   **I am Feeling:**
                                                                   😀 🙂 😐 🙁

How will I make Tommorrow Awesome:

_____
_____

"What you think, you become."
– Buddha

Date: _____ / _____ / _____   Day 5

Breakfast: Lunch: Dinner:

_____   _____   _____
_____   _____   _____
_____   _____   _____
_____   _____   _____

Snacks: Cravings / Response:

_____   _____
_____   _____
_____   _____
_____   _____

Calories   Calories   Water Intake:
Consumed: _____   Burned: _____

Exercise/Workout/Activity:

_____
_____
_____
_____

Weight: _____   Sleep Time: _____   I am Feeling:

How will I make Tommorrow Awesome:

_____
_____

"The journey of a thousand miles begins with one step."
– Lao Tzu

Date: _____/ _____/ _____   Day ⬡ 6

Breakfast: Lunch: Dinner:
_____   _____   _____
_____   _____   _____
_____   _____   _____
_____   _____   _____

Snacks: Cravings / Response:
_____   _____
_____   _____
_____   _____
_____   _____

Calories   Calories   Water Intake:
Consumed: _____   Burned: _____   🥛 🥛 🥛 🥛 🥛

Exercise/Workout/Activity: 🥛 🥛 🥛 🥛 🥛
_____
_____
_____
_____
_____

Weight: _____   Sleep Time: _____   I am Feeling:
                                                         😀 🙂 😐 🙁
How will I make Tommorrow Awesome:
_____
_____

"Do something today that your future self will thank you for."
— Sean Patrick Flanery

Date: _____ / _____ / _____   Day ⬡ 7

Breakfast: Lunch: Dinner:

_____   _____   _____
_____   _____   _____
_____   _____   _____
_____   _____   _____

Snacks: Cravings / Response:

_____   _____
_____   _____
_____   _____
_____   _____

Calories   Calories   Water Intake:
Consumed: _____   Burned: _____

Exercise/Workout/Activity:

_____
_____
_____
_____

Weight: _____   Sleep Time: _____   I am Feeling:
                                                      😀 🙂 😐 🙁

How will I make Tommorrow Awesome:

_____
_____

"Make each day your masterpiece."
– John Wooden

Measurements:

1. Chest: _____
2. Waist: _____
3. Hips: _____
4. Thigh: _____
5. Calf: _____
6. Arm: _____

Weekly Meal Plan:

Weekly Goals: WEEK 2

_____

_____

_____

How I feel about:

Diet: 😃 🙂 😐 🙁

Exercise: 😃 🙂 😐 🙁

Monday: _____
_____

Tuesday: _____
_____

Wednesday: _____
_____

Thursday: _____
_____

Friday: _____
_____

Saturday: _____
_____

Sunday: _____
_____

Notes: _____
_____

Date: _____ / _____ / _____   Day 8

Breakfast: Lunch: Dinner:

_____   _____   _____
_____   _____   _____
_____   _____   _____
_____   _____   _____

Snacks: Cravings / Response:

_____   _____
_____   _____
_____   _____
_____   _____

Calories   Calories   Water Intake:
Consumed: _____   Burned: _____

Exercise/Workout/Activity:

_____
_____
_____
_____

Weight: _____   Sleep Time: _____   I am Feeling:

How will I make Tommorrow Awesome:

_____
_____

"All great achievements require time."
—Maya Angelou

Date: _____ / _____ / _____   Day ⬡ 9

Breakfast: Lunch: Dinner:
_____   _____   _____
_____   _____   _____
_____   _____   _____
_____   _____   _____

Snacks: Cravings / Response:
_____   _____
_____   _____
_____   _____
_____   _____

Calories   Calories   Water Intake:
Consumed: _____   Burned: _____

Exercise/Workout/Activity:
_____
_____
_____
_____
_____

Weight: _____   Sleep Time: _____   I am Feeling:
                                                😀 🙂 😐 🙁
How will I make Tommorrow Awesome:
_____
_____

"Success is going from failure to failure
without losing your enthusiasm."
– Winston Churchill

Date: ____ / ____ / _____

Day 10

Breakfast:

_____

_____

_____

_____

Lunch:

_____

_____

_____

Dinner:

_____

_____

_____

_____

Snacks:

_____

_____

_____

_____

Cravings / Response:

_____

_____

_____

Calories Consumed: _____

Calories Burned: _____

Water Intake:

Exercise/Workout/Activity:

_____

_____

_____

_____

_____

Weight: _____

Sleep Time: _____

I am Feeling:

How will I make Tommorrow Awesome:

_____

_____

*"It's going to be a journey.
It's not a sprint to get in shape."*
—Kerri Walsh Jennings

Date: _____ / _____ / _____   Day ⬡ 11

Breakfast: **Lunch:**   **Dinner:**

_____   _____   _____

_____   _____   _____

_____   _____   _____

_____   _____   _____

Snacks: **Cravings / Response:**

_____   _____

_____   _____

_____   _____

_____   _____

Calories Consumed: _____   **Calories Burned:** _____   **Water Intake:**

Exercise/Workout/Activity:

_____

_____

_____

_____

Weight: _____   **Sleep Time:** _____   **I am Feeling:**

😃 🙂 😐 🙁

How will I make Tommorrow Awesome:

_____

_____

"Inhale the future.
Exhale the past."
–Unknown

Date: _____/ _____/ _____   Day 12

Breakfast: Lunch: Dinner:

_____   _____   _____
_____   _____   _____
_____   _____   _____
_____   _____   _____

Snacks: Cravings / Response:

_____   _____
_____   _____
_____   _____
_____   _____

Calories   Calories   Water Intake:
Consumed: _____   Burned: _____   🥛 🥛 🥛 🥛 🥛
                                                 🥛 🥛 🥛 🥛 🥛
Exercise/Workout/Activity:

_____
_____
_____
_____
_____

Weight: _____   Sleep Time: _____   I am Feeling:
                                                  😃 🙂 😐 🙁
How will I make Tommorrow Awesome:

_____
_____

"You cannot always control what goes on outside,
but you can always control what goes on inside."
–Wayne Dyer

Date: _____/ _____/ _____   Day ⬡ 13

Breakfast: Lunch: Dinner:

_____   _____   _____

_____   _____   _____

_____   _____   _____

_____   _____   _____

Snacks: Cravings / Response:

_____   _____

_____   _____

_____   _____

_____   _____

Calories   Calories   Water Intake:
Consumed: _____   Burned: _____

Exercise/Workout/Activity:

_____

_____

_____

_____

Weight: _____   Sleep Time: _____   I am Feeling:
                                                     😃 🙂 😐 🙁
How will I make Tommorrow Awesome:

_____

_____

"The pain you feel today will be the strength you feel tomorrow."
– Arnold Schwarzenegger

Date: ____ / ____ / _____   Day ⬡ 14

Breakfast: Lunch: Dinner:

_____   _____   _____

_____   _____   _____

_____   _____   _____

_____   _____   _____

Snacks: Cravings / Response:

_____   _____

_____   _____

_____   _____

_____   _____

Calories   Calories   Water Intake:
Consumed: _____   Burned: _____

Exercise/Workout/Activity:

_____

_____

_____

_____

Weight: _____   Sleep Time: _____   I am Feeling:
                                                    😃 🙂 😐 🙁
How will I make Tommorrow Awesome:

_____

_____

"Take care of your body. It's the only place you have to live."
— Jim Rohn

Measurements:

1. Chest: _____
2. Waist: _____
3. Hips: _____
4. Thigh: _____
5. Calf: _____
6. Arm: _____

Weekly Meal Plan:

Weekly Goals: WEEK 3

_____

_____

_____

How I feel about:

Diet: :D :) :| :(

Exercise: :D :) :| :(

Monday:
_____
_____

Tuesday:
_____
_____

Wednesday:
_____
_____

Thursday:
_____
_____

Friday:
_____
_____

Saturday:
_____
_____

Sunday:
_____
_____

Notes:
_____
_____

Date: _____ / _____ / _____   Day 15

Breakfast: Lunch: Dinner:

_____   _____   _____
_____   _____   _____
_____   _____   _____
_____   _____   _____

Snacks: Cravings / Response:

_____   _____
_____   _____
_____   _____
_____   _____

Calories   Calories   Water Intake:
Consumed: _____   Burned: _____

Exercise/Workout/Activity:

_____
_____
_____
_____

Weight: _____   Sleep Time: _____   I am Feeling:

How will I make Tommorrow Awesome:

_____
_____

"Set your goals high, and don't stop till you get there."
– Bo Jackson

Date: _____ / _____ / _____   Day ⬡16

Breakfast: Lunch: Dinner:

_____   _____   _____

_____   _____   _____

_____   _____   _____

_____   _____   _____

Snacks: Cravings / Response:

_____   _____

_____   _____

_____   _____

_____   _____

Calories   Calories   Water Intake:
Consumed: _____   Burned: _____   ⬜⬜⬜⬜⬜⬜
                                                         ⬜⬜⬜⬜⬜⬜
Exercise/Workout/Activity:

_____

_____

_____

_____

Weight: _____   Sleep Time: _____   I am Feeling:
                                                         😃 🙂 😐 ☹️
How will I make Tommorrow Awesome:

_____

_____

*"Just keep going.
Everybody gets better if they keep at it."*
– Ted Williams

Date: _____ / _____ / _____   Day ⬡ 17

Breakfast: Lunch: Dinner:

_____   _____   _____
_____   _____   _____
_____   _____   _____
                                                   _____

Snacks: Cravings / Response:

_____   _____
_____   _____
_____   _____
_____   _____

Calories   Calories   Water Intake:
Consumed: _____   Burned: _____

Exercise/Workout/Activity:

_____
_____
_____
_____
_____

Weight: _____   Sleep Time: _____   I am Feeling:
                                                         ☺ ☺ ☺ ☹
How will I make Tommorrow Awesome:

_____
_____

"Don't limit your challenges, challenge your limits."
– Jerry Dunn

Date: _____/ _____/ _____   Day (18)

Breakfast: Lunch: Dinner:

_____   _____   _____

_____   _____   _____

_____   _____   _____

_____   _____   _____

Snacks: Cravings / Response:

_____   _____

_____   _____

_____   _____

_____   _____

Calories   Calories   Water Intake:
Consumed: _____   Burned: _____

Exercise/Workout/Activity:

_____

_____

_____

_____

Weight: _____   Sleep Time: _____   I am Feeling:

How will I make Tommorrow Awesome:

_____

_____

"Train hard, turn up,
run your best and the rest will take care of itself."
– Usain Bolt

Date: _____ / _____ / _____

Day 19

Breakfast:

_____

_____

_____

_____

Lunch:

_____

_____

_____

_____

Dinner:

_____

_____

_____

_____

Snacks:

_____

_____

_____

_____

Cravings / Response:

_____

_____

_____

_____

Calories Consumed: _____

Calories Burned: _____

Water Intake:

Exercise/Workout/Activity:

_____

_____

_____

_____

Weight: _____

Sleep Time: _____

I am Feeling:

😀 🙂 😐 🙁

How will I make Tommorrow Awesome:

_____

_____

*"Success is walking from failure to failure
with no loss of enthusiasm."*
— Winston Churchill

Date: ____/ ____/ _____   Day 20

Breakfast: Lunch: Dinner:
_____   _____   _____
_____   _____   _____
_____   _____   _____
_____   _____   _____

Snacks: Cravings / Response:
_____   _____
_____   _____
_____   _____
_____   _____

Calories   Calories   Water Intake:
Consumed: _____   Burned: _____

Exercise/Workout/Activity:
_____
_____
_____
_____
_____

Weight: _____   Sleep Time: _____   I am Feeling:
                                                    😀 🙂 😐 🙁
How will I make Tommorrow Awesome:
_____
_____

"If you push me towards a weakness,
I will turn that weakness into a strength."
– Michael Jordan

Date: ____ / ____ / _____   Day ⟨21⟩

Breakfast: Lunch: Dinner:
_____   _____   _____
_____   _____   _____
_____   _____   _____
_____   _____   _____

Snacks: Cravings / Response:
_____   _____
_____   _____
_____   _____
_____   _____

Calories   Calories   Water Intake:
Consumed: _____   Burned: _____   ▭ ▭ ▭ ▭ ▭ ▭
                                                ▭ ▭ ▭ ▭ ▭ ▭
Exercise/Workout/Activity:
_____
_____
_____
_____
_____

Weight: _____   Sleep Time: _____   I am Feeling:
                                                😄 🙂 😐 🙁
How will I make Tommorrow Awesome:
_____
_____

"What to do with a mistake:
recognize it, admit it, learn from it, forget it." – Dean Smith

Measurements:

1. Chest: _____
2. Waist: _____
3. Hips: _____
4. Thigh: _____
5. Calf: _____
6. Arm: _____

Weekly Meal Plan:

Weekly Goals:

_____
_____
_____

How I feel about:

Diet: 😄 🙂 😐 🙁

Exercise: 😄 🙂 😐 🙁

Monday: _____
_____
_____

Tuesday: _____
_____
_____

Wednesday: _____
_____
_____

Thursday: _____
_____
_____

Friday: _____
_____
_____

Saturday: _____
_____
_____

Sunday: _____
_____
_____

Notes: _____
_____
_____

Date: ____/ ____/ _____   Day 22

Breakfast: Lunch: Dinner:

_____   _____   _____
_____   _____   _____
_____   _____   _____
_____   _____   _____

Snacks: Cravings / Response:

_____   _____
_____   _____
_____   _____
_____   _____

Calories   Calories   Water Intake:
Consumed: _____   Burned: _____

Exercise/Workout/Activity:

_____
_____
_____
_____

Weight: _____   Sleep Time: _____   I am Feeling:

How will I make Tommorrow Awesome:

_____
_____

"Good, better, best. Never let it rest.
Until your good is better and your better is best."
— Tim Duncan

Date: _____ / _____ / _____   Day ⬡ 23

Breakfast:
_____
_____
_____
_____

Lunch:
_____
_____
_____
_____

Dinner:
_____
_____
_____
_____

Snacks:
_____
_____
_____
_____

Cravings / Response:
_____
_____
_____
_____

Calories
Consumed: _____

Calories
Burned: _____

Water Intake:

Exercise/Workout/Activity:
_____
_____
_____
_____
_____

Weight: _____   Sleep Time: _____   I am Feeling:
😃 🙂 😐 🙁

How will I make Tommorrow Awesome:
_____
_____

"The future depends on what we do in the present."
–Mahatma Gandhi

Date: _____ / _____ / _____

Day 24

Breakfast:

_____

_____

_____

_____

Lunch:

_____

_____

_____

_____

Dinner:

_____

_____

_____

_____

Snacks:

_____

_____

_____

_____

Cravings / Response:

_____

_____

_____

_____

Calories
Consumed: _____

Calories
Burned: _____

Water Intake:

Exercise/Workout/Activity:

_____

_____

_____

_____

Weight: _____

Sleep Time: _____

I am Feeling:

😃 🙂 😐 🙁

How will I make Tommorrow Awesome:

_____

_____

"Never give up!
Failure and rejection are only the first step to succeeding."
– Jim Valvano

Date: _____/ _____/ _____

Day ⬡ 25

Breakfast:

_____

_____

_____

_____

Lunch:

_____

_____

_____

_____

Dinner:

_____

_____

_____

_____

Snacks:

_____

_____

_____

_____

Cravings / Response:

_____

_____

_____

_____

Calories
Consumed: _____

Calories
Burned: _____

Water Intake:

Exercise/Workout/Activity:

_____

_____

_____

_____

Weight: _____   Sleep Time: _____   I am Feeling:

😀 🙂 😐 🙁

How will I make Tommorrow Awesome:

_____

_____

"It's hard to beat a person who never gives up."
– Babe Ruth

Date: ____ / ____ / _____

Day 26

Breakfast:

Lunch:

Dinner:

_____

_____

_____

_____

Snacks:

Cravings / Response:

Calories Consumed: _____

Calories Burned: _____

Water Intake:

Exercise/Workout/Activity:

Weight: _____

Sleep Time: _____

I am Feeling:

How will I make Tommorrow Awesome:

"Without self-discipline, success is impossible, period."
– Lou Holtz

Date: _____ / _____ / _____   Day ⟨27⟩

Breakfast: Lunch: Dinner:

_____   _____   _____

_____   _____   _____

_____   _____   _____

_____   _____   _____

Snacks: Cravings / Response:

_____   _____

_____   _____

_____   _____

_____   _____

Calories   Calories   Water Intake:
Consumed: _____   Burned: _____

Exercise/Workout/Activity:

_____

_____

_____

_____

_____

Weight: _____   Sleep Time: _____   I am Feeling:

                                                        😃 🙂 😐 🙁

How will I make Tommorrow Awesome:

_____

_____

*"Never let your head hang down.
Never give up and sit down and grieve. Find another way."
– Satchel Paige*

Date: _____ / _____ / _____   Day 28

Breakfast: Lunch: Dinner:

_____   _____   _____
_____   _____   _____
_____   _____   _____
_____   _____   _____

Snacks: Cravings / Response:

_____   _____
_____   _____
_____   _____
_____   _____

Calories   Calories   Water Intake:
Consumed: _____   Burned: _____

Exercise/Workout/Activity:

_____
_____
_____
_____

Weight: _____   Sleep Time: _____   I am Feeling:
                                                     😄 🙂 😐 🙁
How will I make Tommorow Awesome:

_____
_____

"You're only one workout away from a good mood."
– Unknown

Measurements:

1. Chest: _____
2. Waist: _____
3. Hips: _____
4. Thigh: _____
5. Calf: _____
6. Arm: _____

Weekly Meal Plan:

Monday: _____
_____
_____

Tuesday: _____
_____
_____

Wednesday: _____
_____
_____

Thursday: _____
_____
_____

Friday: _____
_____
_____

Saturday: _____
_____
_____

Sunday: _____
_____
_____

Notes: _____
_____
_____

Weekly Goals: WEEK 5

_____
_____
_____

How I feel about:

Diet: 😃 🙂 😐 🙁

Exercise: 😃 🙂 😐 🙁

Date: _____ / _____ / _____   Day 29

Breakfast: Lunch: Dinner:
_____   _____   _____
_____   _____   _____
_____   _____   _____
_____   _____   _____

Snacks: Cravings / Response:
_____   _____
_____   _____
_____   _____
_____   _____

Calories   Calories   Water Intake:
Consumed: _____   Burned: _____

Exercise/Workout/Activity:
_____
_____
_____
_____

Weight: _____   Sleep Time: _____   I am Feeling:

How will I make Tommorrow Awesome:
_____
_____

"If you can believe it, the mind can achieve it."
– Ronnie Lott

Date: _____/ _____/ _____   Day ⬡30

Breakfast: Lunch: Dinner:

_____   _____   _____
_____   _____   _____
_____   _____   _____
_____   _____   _____

Snacks: Cravings / Response:

_____   _____
_____   _____
_____   _____
_____   _____

Calories   Calories   Water Intake:
Consumed: _____   Burned: _____

Exercise/Workout/Activity:

_____
_____
_____
_____
_____

Weight: _____   Sleep Time: _____   I am Feeling:
                                                   😃 🙂 😐 🙁
How will I make Tommorrow Awesome:

_____
_____

"Push yourself again and again.
Don't give an inch until the final buzzer sounds."
– Larry Bird

Date: ____ / ____ / _____

Day 31

Breakfast:
_____
_____
_____
_____

Lunch:
_____
_____
_____

Dinner:
_____
_____
_____
_____

Snacks:
_____
_____
_____
_____

Cravings / Response:
_____
_____
_____

Calories
Consumed: _____

Calories
Burned: _____

Water Intake:

Exercise/Workout/Activity:
_____
_____
_____
_____

Weight: _____

Sleep Time: _____

I am Feeling:

😃 😊 😐 🙁

How will I make Tommorrow Awesome:
_____
_____

"If you aren't going all the way, why go at all?"
– Joe Namath

Date: _____/ _____/ _____   Day ⬡ 32

Breakfast: Lunch: Dinner:
_____   _____   _____
_____   _____   _____
_____   _____   _____
_____   _____   _____

Snacks: Cravings / Response:
_____   _____
_____   _____
_____   _____
_____   _____

Calories   Calories   Water Intake:
Consumed: _____   Burned: _____   🥛🥛🥛🥛🥛
                                                      🥛🥛🥛🥛🥛
Exercise/Workout/Activity:
_____
_____
_____
_____

Weight: _____   Sleep Time: _____   I am Feeling:
                                                      😃 🙂 😐 🙁
How will I make Tommorrow Awesome:
_____
_____

"Age is no barrier. It's a limitation you put on your mind."
– Jackie Joyner-Kersee

Date: ____ / ____ / _____

Day 33

Breakfast:

_____

_____

_____

_____

Lunch:

_____

_____

_____

_____

Dinner:

_____

_____

_____

_____

Snacks:

_____

_____

_____

_____

Cravings / Response:

_____

_____

_____

_____

Calories Consumed: _____

Calories Burned: _____

Water Intake:

Exercise/Workout/Activity:

_____

_____

_____

_____

Weight: _____

Sleep Time: _____

I am Feeling:

How will I make Tommorrow Awesome:

_____

_____

*"The difference between the impossible and the possible
lies in a person's determination."*
– Tommy Lasorda

Date: _____ / _____ / _____

Day (34)

Breakfast:

_____

_____

_____

_____

Lunch:

_____

_____

_____

_____

Dinner:

_____

_____

_____

_____

Snacks:

_____

_____

_____

_____

Cravings / Response:

_____

_____

_____

_____

Calories
Consumed: _____

Calories
Burned: _____

Water Intake:

Exercise/Workout/Activity:

_____

_____

_____

_____

_____

Weight: _____

Sleep Time: _____

I am Feeling:

😄 🙂 😐 🙁

How will I make Tommorrow Awesome:

_____

_____

"Do what you have to do until you can do what you want to do."
– Oprah Winfrey

Date: ____/ ____/ _____   Day 35

Breakfast: Lunch: Dinner:
_____   _____   _____
_____   _____   _____
_____   _____   _____
_____   _____   _____

Snacks: Cravings / Response:
_____   _____
_____   _____
_____   _____
_____   _____

Calories   Calories   Water Intake:
Consumed: _____   Burned: _____

Exercise/Workout/Activity:
_____
_____
_____
_____

Weight: _____   Sleep Time: _____   I am Feeling:

How will I make Tommorow Awesome:
_____
_____

"I've learned that something constructive comes from every defeat."
– Tom Landry

Measurements:

1. Chest: _____
2. Waist: _____
3. Hips: _____
4. Thigh: _____
5. Calf: _____
6. Arm: _____

Weekly Meal Plan:

Weekly Goals: WEEK 6

_____

_____

_____

How I feel about:

Diet: 😃 🙂 😐 🙁

Exercise: 😃 🙂 😐 🙁

Monday:
_____
_____

Tuesday:
_____
_____

Wednesday:
_____
_____

Thursday:
_____
_____

Friday:
_____
_____

Saturday:
_____
_____

Sunday:
_____
_____

Notes:
_____
_____

Date: _____ / _____ / _____

Day 36

Breakfast:

_____
_____
_____
_____

Lunch:

_____
_____
_____
_____

Dinner:

_____
_____
_____
_____

Snacks:

_____
_____
_____
_____

Cravings / Response:

_____
_____
_____
_____

Calories Consumed: _____

Calories Burned: _____

Water Intake:

Exercise/Workout/Activity:

_____
_____
_____
_____

Weight: _____

Sleep Time: _____

I am Feeling:

How will I make Tommorrow Awesome:

_____
_____

*"Make sure your worst enemy doesn't live
between your own two ears."*
– Laird Hamilton

Date: ____ / ____ / _____

Day 37

Breakfast:

_____

_____

_____

_____

Lunch:

_____

_____

_____

_____

Dinner:

_____

_____

_____

_____

Snacks:

_____

_____

_____

_____

Cravings / Response:

_____

_____

_____

_____

Calories
Consumed: _____

Calories
Burned: _____

Water Intake:

Exercise/Workout/Activity:

_____

_____

_____

_____

_____

Weight: _____

Sleep Time: _____

I am Feeling:
😃 🙂 😐 🙁

How will I make Tommorrow Awesome:

_____

_____

"The will to win is important, but the will to prepare is vital."
– Joe Paterno

Date: _____ / _____ / _____   Day 38

Breakfast: **Lunch:**   **Dinner:**
_____   _____   _____
_____   _____   _____
_____   _____   _____
_____   _____   _____

Snacks: **Cravings / Response:**
_____   _____
_____   _____
_____   _____
_____   _____

Calories   **Calories**   **Water Intake:**
Consumed: _____   **Burned:** _____

Exercise/Workout/Activity:
_____
_____
_____
_____

Weight: _____   **Sleep Time:** _____   **I am Feeling:**

How will I make Tommorrow Awesome:
_____
_____

"You're never a loser until you quit trying."
– Mike Ditka

Date: _____ / _____ / _____   Day 39

Breakfast: Lunch: Dinner:

_____   _____   _____
_____   _____   _____
_____   _____   _____
_____   _____   _____

Snacks: Cravings / Response:

_____   _____
_____   _____
_____   _____
_____   _____

Calories   Calories   Water Intake:
Consumed: _____   Burned: _____

Exercise/Workout/Activity:

_____
_____
_____
_____

Weight: _____   Sleep Time: _____   I am Feeling:
                                                     :) :) :| :(

How will I make Tommorrow Awesome:

_____
_____

*"It's not whether you get knocked down;
it's whether you get up."
– Vince Lombardi*

Date: _____ / _____ / _____

Day 40

Breakfast:

Lunch:

Dinner:

_____
_____
_____
_____

_____
_____
_____
_____

_____
_____
_____
_____

Snacks:

Cravings / Response:

_____
_____
_____

_____
_____
_____

Calories
Consumed: _____

Calories
Burned: _____

Water Intake:

Exercise/Workout/Activity:

_____
_____
_____
_____

Weight: _____

Sleep Time: _____

I am Feeling:

😃 🙂 😐 🙁

How will I make Tommorrow Awesome:

_____
_____

"Today I will do what others won't,
so tomorrow I can accomplish what others can't."
– Jerry Rice

Date: _____ / _____ / _____   Day ⬡41⬡

Breakfast: Lunch: Dinner:

_____   _____   _____

_____   _____   _____

_____   _____   _____

_____   _____   _____

Snacks: Cravings / Response:

_____   _____

_____   _____

_____   _____

Calories   Calories   Water Intake:
Consumed: _____   Burned: _____   🥛🥛🥛🥛🥛

Exercise/Workout/Activity: 🥛🥛🥛🥛🥛

_____

_____

_____

_____

Weight: _____   Sleep Time: _____   I am Feeling:

                                                         😃 😊 😐 ☹️

How will I make Tommorrow Awesome:

_____

_____

"The more difficult the victory,
the greater the happiness in winning."
– Pele

Date: _____ / _____ / _____

Day 42

Breakfast:

_____
_____
_____
_____

Lunch:

_____
_____
_____
_____

Dinner:

_____
_____
_____
_____

Snacks:

_____
_____
_____
_____

Cravings / Response:

_____
_____
_____
_____

Calories Consumed: _____

Calories Burned: _____

Water Intake:

Exercise/Workout/Activity:

_____
_____
_____
_____

Weight: _____

Sleep Time: _____

I am Feeling:

How will I make Tommorrow Awesome:

_____
_____

"Everything is practice."
– Bill Shankley

Measurements:

1. Chest: _____
2. Waist: _____
3. Hips: _____
4. Thigh: _____
5. Calf: _____
6. Arm: _____

Weekly Meal Plan:

Weekly Goals:

_____
_____
_____

How I feel about:

Diet: 😀 🙂 😐 ☹️

Exercise: 😀 🙂 😐 ☹️

Monday:
_____
_____

Tuesday:
_____
_____

Wednesday:
_____
_____

Thursday:
_____
_____

Friday:
_____
_____

Saturday:
_____
_____

Sunday:
_____
_____

Notes:
_____
_____

Date: ____ / ____ / _____

Day 43

Breakfast:

_____
_____
_____
_____

Lunch:

_____
_____
_____
_____

Dinner:

_____
_____
_____
_____

Snacks:

_____
_____
_____
_____

Cravings / Response:

_____
_____
_____
_____

Calories Consumed: _____

Calories Burned: _____

Water Intake:

Exercise/Workout/Activity:

_____
_____
_____
_____

Weight: _____

Sleep Time: _____

I am Feeling:

How will I make Tommorrow Awesome:

_____
_____

"A champion is someone who gets up when he can't."
– Jack Dempsey

Date: ____/ ____/ _____   Day 44

Breakfast: Lunch: Dinner:

_____   _____   _____

_____   _____   _____

_____   _____   _____

_____   _____   _____

Snacks: Cravings / Response:

_____   _____

_____   _____

_____   _____

_____   _____

Calories   Calories   Water Intake:
Consumed: _____   Burned: _____

Exercise/Workout/Activity:

_____

_____

_____

_____

Weight: _____   Sleep Time: _____   I am Feeling:

                                                    😀 🙂 😐 🙁

How will I make Tommorrow Awesome:

_____

_____

"Do something today that your future self will thank you for."
– Unknown

Date: _____ / _____ / _____

Day 45

Breakfast:

_____
_____
_____
_____

Lunch:

_____
_____
_____
_____

Dinner:

_____
_____
_____
_____

Snacks:

_____
_____
_____

Cravings / Response:

_____
_____
_____
_____

Calories Consumed: _____

Calories Burned: _____

Water Intake:

Exercise/Workout/Activity:

_____
_____
_____
_____

Weight: _____

Sleep Time: _____

I am Feeling:

How will I make Tommorrow Awesome:

_____
_____

"You miss 100% of the shots you don't take."
– Wayne Gretzky

Date: _____/ _____/ _____   Day ⬡ 46

Breakfast: Lunch: Dinner:

_____   _____   _____

_____   _____   _____

_____   _____   _____

_____   _____   _____

Snacks: Cravings / Response:

_____   _____

_____   _____

_____   _____

_____   _____

Calories   Calories   Water Intake:
Consumed: _____   Burned: _____
                                                    🥛🥛🥛🥛🥛
Exercise/Workout/Activity: 🥛🥛🥛🥛🥛

_____

_____

_____

_____

Weight: _____   Sleep Time: _____   I am Feeling:

                                                    😀 🙂 😐 🙁

How will I make Tommorrow Awesome:

_____

_____

"What hurts today makes you stronger tomorrow."
– Jay Cutler

Date: _____ / _____ / _____

Day 47

Breakfast:

_____
_____
_____
_____

Lunch:

_____
_____
_____
_____

Dinner:

_____
_____
_____
_____

Snacks:

_____
_____
_____
_____

Cravings / Response:

_____
_____
_____
_____

Calories Consumed: _____

Calories Burned: _____

Water Intake:

Exercise/Workout/Activity:

_____
_____
_____
_____

Weight: _____

Sleep Time: _____

I am Feeling:

😃 🙂 😐 🙁

How will I make Tommorrow Awesome:

_____

*"This ability to conquer oneself is no doubt
the most precious of all things sports bestows."*
– Olga Korbut

Date: ____ / ____ / _____

Day 48

Breakfast:

_____
_____
_____
_____

Lunch:

_____
_____
_____
_____

Dinner:

_____
_____
_____
_____

Snacks:

_____
_____
_____
_____

Cravings / Response:

_____
_____
_____
_____

Calories Consumed: _____

Calories Burned: _____

Water Intake:

Exercise/Workout/Activity:

_____
_____
_____
_____
_____

Weight: _____

Sleep Time: _____

I am Feeling:

How will I make Tommorrow Awesome:

_____
_____

"Strength does not come from physical capacity.
It comes from an indomitable will."
– Mahatma Gandhi

Date: _____ / _____ / _____   Day (49)

Breakfast: Lunch: Dinner:
_____   _____   _____
_____   _____   _____
_____   _____   _____
_____   _____   _____

Snacks: Cravings / Response:
_____   _____
_____   _____
_____   _____
_____   _____

Calories   Calories   Water Intake:
Consumed: _____   Burned: _____

Exercise/Workout/Activity:
_____
_____
_____
_____
_____

Weight: _____   Sleep Time: _____   I am Feeling:

How will I make Tommorrow Awesome:
_____
_____

"He who is not courageous enough to take risks
will accomplish nothing in life."
– Muhammad Ali

Measurements:

1. Chest: _____

2. Waist: _____

3. Hips: _____

4. Thigh: _____

5. Calf: _____

6. Arm: _____

Weekly Meal Plan:

Weekly Goals:

_____

_____

_____

How I feel about:

Diet: 😃 🙂 😐 🙁

Exercise: 😃 🙂 😐 🙁

Monday:
_____
_____

Tuesday:
_____
_____

Wednesday:
_____
_____

Thursday:
_____
_____

Friday:
_____
_____

Saturday:
_____
_____

Sunday:
_____
_____

Notes:
_____
_____

Date: _____ / _____ / _____

Breakfast:

Lunch:

Dinner:

Snacks:

Cravings / Response:

Calories Consumed: _____

Calories Burned: _____

Water Intake:

Exercise/Workout/Activity:

Weight: _____

Sleep Time: _____

I am Feeling:

How will I make Tommorrow Awesome:

"It is more difficult to stay on top than to get there."
– Mia Hamm

Date: _____/ _____/ _____

Breakfast:

_____

_____

_____

_____

Lunch:

_____

_____

_____

_____

Dinner:

_____

_____

_____

_____

Snacks:

_____

_____

_____

_____

Cravings / Response:

_____

_____

_____

_____

Calories
Consumed: _____

Calories
Burned: _____

Water Intake:

Exercise/Workout/Activity:

_____

_____

_____

_____

Weight: _____

Sleep Time: _____

I am Feeling:

How will I make Tommorrow Awesome:

_____

_____

*"All our dreams can come true
if we have the courage to pursue them."*
– Walt Disney

Date: _____ / _____ / _____   Day ⬡52

Breakfast: **Lunch:**   **Dinner:**
_____   _____   _____
_____   _____   _____
_____   _____   _____
_____   _____   _____

Snacks: **Cravings / Response:**
_____   _____
_____   _____
_____   _____
_____   _____

Calories   **Calories**   Water Intake:
Consumed: _____   **Burned:** _____   🥛 🥛 🥛 🥛 🥛

Exercise/Workout/Activity: 🥛 🥛 🥛 🥛 🥛
_____
_____
_____
_____

Weight: _____   **Sleep Time:** _____   I am Feeling:
                                                          😃 🙂 😐 🙁
How will I make Tommorrow Awesome:
_____
_____

"If you want something you've never had,
you must be willing to do something you've never done."
— Thomas Jefferson

Date: ____/ ____/ _____

Day 53

Breakfast:

_____
_____
_____
_____

Lunch:

_____
_____
_____
_____

Dinner:

_____
_____
_____
_____

Snacks:

_____
_____
_____
_____

Cravings / Response:

_____
_____
_____
_____

Calories
Consumed: _____

Calories
Burned: _____

Water Intake:

Exercise/Workout/Activity:

_____
_____
_____
_____
_____

Weight: _____   Sleep Time: _____   I am Feeling:

How will I make Tommorrow Awesome:

_____
_____

"The difference between try and triumph is a little 'umph'."
– Unknown

Date: _____ / _____ / _____

Day 54

Breakfast:

Lunch:

Dinner:

_____

_____

_____

_____

_____

_____

_____

_____

_____

_____

Snacks:

Cravings / Response:

_____

_____

_____

_____

_____

_____

_____

_____

Calories Consumed: _____

Calories Burned: _____

Water Intake:

Exercise/Workout/Activity:

_____

_____

_____

_____

_____

Weight: _____

Sleep Time: _____

I am Feeling:

How will I make Tommorrow Awesome:

_____

_____

"You have to think it before you can do it.
The mind is what makes it all possible."
– Kai Greene

Date: ____/ ____/ _____   Day 55

Breakfast: Lunch: Dinner:
_____   _____   _____
_____   _____   _____
_____   _____   _____
_____   _____   _____

Snacks: Cravings / Response:
_____   _____
_____   _____
_____   _____
_____   _____

Calories   Calories   Water Intake:
Consumed: _____   Burned: _____   [glasses icons]

Exercise/Workout/Activity: [glasses icons]
_____
_____
_____
_____
_____

Weight: _____   Sleep Time: _____   I am Feeling:
                                                     ☺ ☺ ☻ ☹
How will I make Tommorrow Awesome:
_____
_____

*"If you have everything under control,
you're not moving fast enough."
– Mario Andretti*

Date: _____ / _____ / _____   Day 56

Breakfast: Lunch: Dinner:

_____   _____   _____
_____   _____   _____
_____   _____   _____
_____   _____   _____

Snacks: Cravings / Response:

_____   _____
_____   _____
_____   _____
_____   _____

Calories   Calories   Water Intake:
Consumed: _____   Burned: _____

Exercise/Workout/Activity:

_____
_____
_____
_____

Weight: _____   Sleep Time: _____   I am Feeling:

How will I make Tommorrow Awesome:

_____
_____

"Each of us has a fire in our hearts for something.
It's our goal in life to find it and keep it lit."
– Mary Lou Retton

Measurements:

1. Chest: _____
2. Waist: _____
3. Hips: _____
4. Thigh: _____
5. Calf: _____
6. Arm: _____

Weekly Meal Plan:

Weekly Goals:

_____

_____

_____

How I feel about:

Diet: 😀 🙂 😐 🙁

Exercise: 😀 🙂 😐 🙁

Monday: _____

_____

_____

Tuesday: _____

_____

_____

Wednesday: _____

_____

_____

Thursday: _____

_____

_____

Friday: _____

_____

_____

Saturday: _____

_____

_____

Sunday: _____

_____

_____

Notes: _____

_____

_____

Date: _____ / _____ / _____

Day 57

Breakfast:

_____

_____

_____

_____

Lunch:

_____

_____

_____

_____

Dinner:

_____

_____

_____

_____

Snacks:

_____

_____

_____

_____

Cravings / Response:

_____

_____

_____

Calories Consumed: _____

Calories Burned: _____

Water Intake:

Exercise/Workout/Activity:

_____

_____

_____

_____

Weight: _____

Sleep Time: _____

I am Feeling:

How will I make Tommorrow Awesome:

_____

_____

"Mental will is a muscle that needs exercise,
just like muscles of the body."
– Lynn Jennings

Date: ____/ ____/ _____

Day 58

Breakfast:

_____

_____

_____

_____

Lunch:

_____

_____

_____

_____

Dinner:

_____

_____

_____

_____

Snacks:

_____

_____

_____

_____

Cravings / Response:

_____

_____

_____

_____

Calories Consumed: _____

Calories Burned: _____

Water Intake:

Exercise/Workout/Activity:

_____

_____

_____

_____

_____

Weight: _____

Sleep Time: _____

I am Feeling:

How will I make Tommorrow Awesome:

_____

_____

"To give any less than your best is to sacrifice a gift."
– Steve Prefontaine

Date: _____ / _____ / _____

Day 59

Breakfast:

_____

_____

_____

_____

Lunch:

_____

_____

_____

_____

Dinner:

_____

_____

_____

_____

Snacks:

_____

_____

_____

Cravings / Response:

_____

_____

_____

_____

Calories Consumed: _____

Calories Burned: _____

Water Intake:

Exercise/Workout/Activity:

_____

_____

_____

_____

Weight: _____

Sleep Time: _____

I am Feeling:

😃 🙂 😐 🙁

How will I make Tommorrow Awesome:

_____

_____

"What makes something special is not just what you have to gain,
but what you feel there is to lose."
– Andre Agassi

Date: _____ / _____ / _____

Day (60)

Breakfast:

_____

_____

_____

_____

Lunch:

_____

_____

_____

_____

Dinner:

_____

_____

_____

_____

Snacks:

_____

_____

_____

_____

Cravings / Response:

_____

_____

_____

_____

Calories Consumed: _____

Calories Burned: _____

Water Intake:

Exercise/Workout/Activity:

_____

_____

_____

_____

_____

Weight: _____

Sleep Time: _____

I am Feeling:

How will I make Tommorrow Awesome:

_____

_____

"Always make a total effort, even when the odds are against you."
– Arnold Palmer

Date: ____ / ____ / _____

Day 61

Breakfast:

_____
_____
_____
_____

Lunch:

_____
_____
_____
_____

Dinner:

_____
_____
_____
_____

Snacks:

_____
_____
_____

Cravings / Response:

_____
_____
_____
_____

Calories Consumed: _____

Calories Burned: _____

Water Intake:

Exercise/Workout/Activity:

_____
_____
_____
_____

Weight: _____

Sleep Time: _____

I am Feeling:

☺ ☺ ☺ ☹

How will I make Tommorrow Awesome:

_____
_____

"Never underestimate the power of dreams and the influence of the human spirit. The potential for greatness lives within each of us."
– Wilma Rudolph

Date: ____/ ____/ _____   Day 62

Breakfast: Lunch: Dinner:

_____   _____   _____

_____   _____   _____

_____   _____   _____

_____   _____   _____

Snacks: Cravings / Response:

_____   _____

_____   _____

_____   _____

_____   _____

Calories   Calories   Water Intake:
Consumed: _____   Burned: _____

Exercise/Workout/Activity:

_____

_____

_____

_____

_____

Weight: _____   Sleep Time: _____   I am Feeling:

How will I make Tommorrow Awesome:

_____

_____

"Life begins at the end of your comfort zone."
– Unknown

Date: ____ / ____ / _____

Day 63

Breakfast:

_____

_____

_____

_____

Lunch:

_____

_____

_____

_____

Dinner:

_____

_____

_____

_____

Snacks:

_____

_____

_____

Cravings / Response:

_____

_____

_____

Calories
Consumed: _____

Calories
Burned: _____

Water Intake:

Exercise/Workout/Activity:

_____

_____

_____

_____

Weight: _____

Sleep Time: _____

I am Feeling:

How will I make Tommorrow Awesome:

_____

_____

_____

"You have to believe in yourself when no one else does
— that makes you a winner right there."
— Venus Williams

Measurements:

1. Chest: _____
2. Waist: _____
3. Hips: _____
4. Thigh: _____
5. Calf: _____
6. Arm: _____

Weekly Meal Plan:

Weekly Goals: WEEK 10

_____

_____

_____

How I feel about:

Diet: 😃 🙂 😐 🙁

Exercise: 😃 🙂 😐 🙁

Monday: _____

_____

Tuesday: _____

_____

Wednesday: _____

_____

Thursday: _____

_____

Friday: _____

_____

Saturday: _____

_____

Sunday: _____

_____

Notes: _____

_____

Date: ____ / ____ / _____

Day 64

Breakfast:
_____
_____
_____
_____

Lunch:
_____
_____
_____
_____

Dinner:
_____
_____
_____
_____

Snacks:
_____
_____
_____
_____

Cravings / Response:
_____
_____
_____
_____

Calories Consumed: _____

Calories Burned: _____

Water Intake:

Exercise/Workout/Activity:
_____
_____
_____
_____
_____

Weight: _____

Sleep Time: _____

I am Feeling:

How will I make Tommorrow Awesome:
_____
_____

"Run when you can, walk if you have to,
crawl if you must; just never give up."
– Dean Karnazes

Date: _____/ _____/ _____

Day 65

Breakfast:

_____
_____
_____
_____

Lunch:

_____
_____
_____
_____

Dinner:

_____
_____
_____
_____

Snacks:

_____
_____
_____

Cravings / Response:

_____
_____
_____
_____

Calories Consumed: _____

Calories Burned: _____

Water Intake:

Exercise/Workout/Activity:

_____
_____
_____
_____
_____

Weight: _____   Sleep Time: _____   I am Feeling:

How will I make Tommorrow Awesome:

_____
_____

*"We must train hard. It's not about denying a weakness
may exist but about denying its right to persist."*
– Vince McConnell

Date: _____ / _____ / _____

Day 66

Breakfast:
_____
_____
_____
_____

Lunch:
_____
_____
_____

Dinner:
_____
_____
_____

Snacks:
_____
_____
_____

Cravings / Response:
_____
_____
_____

Calories Consumed: _____

Calories Burned: _____

Water Intake:

Exercise/Workout/Activity:
_____
_____
_____
_____

Weight: _____

Sleep Time: _____

I am Feeling:

How will I make Tommorrow Awesome:
_____
_____

"If it doesn't challenge you, it won't change you."
– Fred Devito

Date: ____/ ____/ _____   Day 67

Breakfast: Lunch: Dinner:

_____   _____   _____
_____   _____   _____
_____   _____   _____
_____   _____   _____

Snacks: Cravings / Response:

_____   _____
_____   _____
_____   _____

Calories   Calories   Water Intake:
Consumed: _____   Burned: _____

Exercise/Workout/Activity:

_____
_____
_____
_____

Weight: _____   Sleep Time: _____   I am Feeling:
                                                    😃 🙂 😐 🙁

How will I make Tommorrow Awesome:

_____
_____

*"To uncover your true potential you must first find your own limits
and then you have to have the courage to blow past them."*
– Picabo Street

Date: ____/ ____/ _____

Day 68

Breakfast:

_____

_____

_____

_____

Lunch:

_____

_____

_____

_____

Dinner:

_____

_____

_____

_____

Snacks:

_____

_____

_____

_____

Cravings / Response:

_____

_____

_____

_____

Calories Consumed: _____

Calories Burned: _____

Water Intake:

Exercise/Workout/Activity:

_____

_____

_____

_____

Weight: _____

Sleep Time: _____

I am Feeling:

😃 🙂 😐 🙁

How will I make Tommorrow Awesome:

_____

_____

"If you dream and you allow yourself to dream
you can do anything."
– Clara Hughes

Date: ____ / ____ / _____

Day 69

Breakfast:

_____
_____
_____
_____

Lunch:

_____
_____
_____
_____

Dinner:

_____
_____
_____
_____

Snacks:

_____
_____
_____
_____

Cravings / Response:

_____
_____
_____
_____

Calories Consumed: _____

Calories Burned: _____

Water Intake:

Exercise/Workout/Activity:

_____
_____
_____
_____
_____

Weight: _____

Sleep Time: _____

I am Feeling:

How will I make Tommorrow Awesome:

_____
_____

"Strength does not come from winning.
Your struggles develop your strengths."
– Arnold Schwarzenegger

Date: _____ / _____ / _____

Breakfast:

_____

_____

_____

_____

Lunch:

_____

_____

_____

_____

Dinner:

_____

_____

_____

_____

Snacks:

_____

_____

_____

_____

Cravings / Response:

_____

_____

_____

_____

Calories Consumed: _____

Calories Burned: _____

Water Intake:

Exercise/Workout/Activity:

_____

_____

_____

_____

Weight: _____

Sleep Time: _____

I am Feeling:

How will I make Tommorrow Awesome:

_____

_____

"You are the sky, everything else is just the weather."
– Pema Chodron

Measurements:

1. Chest: _____
2. Waist: _____
3. Hips: _____
4. Thigh: _____
5. Calf: _____
6. Arm: _____

Weekly Meal Plan:

Weekly Goals:

_____

_____

_____

How I feel about:

Diet: 😀 🙂 😐 🙁

Exercise: 😀 🙂 😐 🙁

Monday:

Tuesday:

Wednesday:

Thursday:

Friday:

Saturday:

Sunday:

Notes:

Date: ____/ ____/ _____   Day ⬡71⬡

Breakfast: **Lunch:**   **Dinner:**
_____   _____   _____
_____   _____   _____
_____   _____   _____
_____   _____   _____

Snacks: **Cravings / Response:**
_____   _____
_____   _____
_____   _____
_____   _____

Calories   **Calories**   **Water Intake:**
Consumed: _____   **Burned:** _____

Exercise/Workout/Activity:
_____
_____
_____
_____

Weight: _____   **Sleep Time:** _____   **I am Feeling:**

How will I make Tommorrow Awesome:
_____
_____

"It's all about the journey, not the outcome."
– Carl Lewis

Date: _____ / _____ / _____   Day 72

Breakfast: Lunch: Dinner:

_____   _____   _____

_____   _____   _____

_____   _____   _____

_____   _____   _____

Snacks: Cravings / Response:

_____   _____

_____   _____

_____   _____

_____   _____

Calories   Calories   Water Intake:
Consumed: _____   Burned: _____

Exercise/Workout/Activity:

_____

_____

_____

_____

_____

Weight: _____   Sleep Time: _____   I am Feeling:

How will I make Tommorrow Awesome:

_____

_____

The soul is here for its own joy.
– Rumi

Date: _____ / _____ / _____

Day (73)

Breakfast:

_____
_____
_____
_____

Lunch:

_____
_____
_____
_____

Dinner:

_____
_____
_____
_____

Snacks:

_____
_____
_____
_____

Cravings / Response:

_____
_____
_____
_____

Calories
Consumed: _____

Calories
Burned: _____

Water Intake:

Exercise/Workout/Activity:

_____
_____
_____
_____

Weight: _____

Sleep Time: _____

I am Feeling:

😃 🙂 😐 🙁

How will I make Tommorrow Awesome:

_____
_____

"Quitters never win, and winners never quit."
– Unknown

Date: _____ / _____ / _____   Day ⬡74

Breakfast: Lunch: Dinner:

_____   _____   _____

_____   _____   _____

_____   _____   _____

_____   _____   _____

Snacks: Cravings / Response:

_____   _____

_____   _____

_____   _____

_____   _____

Calories   Calories   Water Intake:
Consumed: _____   Burned: _____

Exercise/Workout/Activity:

_____

_____

_____

_____

_____

Weight: _____   Sleep Time: _____   I am Feeling:

                                                          😀 🙂 😐 🙁

How will I make Tommorrow Awesome:

_____

_____

*"Meditation is a way for nourishing and
blossoming the divinity within you."
– Amit Ray*

ate: _____ / _____ / _____   Day (75)

Breakfast: Lunch: Dinner:
_____   _____   _____
_____   _____   _____
_____   _____   _____
_____   _____   _____

Snacks: Cravings / Response:
_____   _____
_____   _____
_____   _____
_____   _____

Calories   Calories   Water Intake:
Consumed: _____   Burned: _____

Exercise/Workout/Activity:
_____
_____
_____
_____

Weight: _____   Sleep Time: _____   I am Feeling:
                                                 😃 🙂 😐 🙁
How will I make Tommorrow Awesome:
_____
_____

"People often say that motivation doesn't last.
Well, neither does bathing. That's why we recommend it daily."
– Zig Ziglar

Date: _____/ _____/ _____

Day 76

Breakfast:

_____
_____
_____
_____

Lunch:

_____
_____
_____
_____

Dinner:

_____
_____
_____
_____

Snacks:

_____
_____
_____
_____

Cravings / Response:

_____
_____
_____
_____

Calories
Consumed: _____

Calories
Burned: _____

Water Intake:

Exercise/Workout/Activity:

_____
_____
_____
_____
_____

Weight: _____

Sleep Time: _____

I am Feeling:

How will I make Tommorrow Awesome:

_____
_____

*"Go confidently in the direction of your dreams.
Live the life you have imagined."*
– Henry David Thoreau

Date: _____/ _____/ _____

Day 77

Breakfast:

Lunch:

Dinner:

_____
_____
_____
_____

_____
_____
_____
_____

_____
_____
_____
_____

Snacks:

Cravings / Response:

_____
_____
_____
_____

_____
_____
_____
_____

Calories
Consumed: _____

Calories
Burned: _____

Water Intake:

Exercise/Workout/Activity:

_____
_____
_____
_____

Weight: _____

Sleep Time: _____

I am Feeling:

How will I make Tommorrow Awesome:

_____
_____

"Life is not measured by the number of breaths we take,
but by the moments that take our breath away."
– Maya Angelou

Measurements:

1. Chest: _____
2. Waist: _____
3. Hips: _____
4. Thigh: _____
5. Calf: _____
6. Arm: _____

Weekly Goals: WEEK 12

_____
_____
_____

How I feel about:

Diet: 😃 🙂 😐 🙁

Exercise: 😃 🙂 😐 🙁

Weekly Meal Plan:

Monday: _____
_____
_____

Tuesday: _____
_____
_____

Wednesday: _____
_____
_____

Thursday: _____
_____
_____

Friday: _____
_____
_____

Saturday: _____
_____
_____

Sunday: _____
_____
_____

Notes: _____
_____
_____

Date: ____/ ____/ _____   Day (78)

Breakfast: Lunch: Dinner:

_____   _____   _____
_____   _____   _____
_____   _____   _____
_____   _____   _____

Snacks: Cravings / Response:

_____   _____
_____   _____
_____   _____
_____   _____

Calories   Calories   Water Intake:
Consumed: _____   Burned: _____   ⬜⬜⬜⬜⬜⬜
                                                       ⬜⬜⬜⬜⬜⬜
Exercise/Workout/Activity:

_____
_____
_____
_____

Weight: _____   Sleep Time: _____   I am Feeling:
                                                       😃 🙂 😐 🙁
How will I make Tommorrow Awesome:

_____
_____

*"There is only one corner of the universe you can be certain
of improving, and that's your own self."*
– Aldous Huxley

Date: ____/ ____/ _____

Day 79

Breakfast:

_____

_____

_____

_____

Lunch:

_____

_____

_____

_____

Dinner:

_____

_____

_____

_____

Snacks:

_____

_____

_____

_____

Cravings / Response:

_____

_____

_____

_____

Calories Consumed: _____

Calories Burned: _____

Water Intake:

Exercise/Workout/Activity:

_____

_____

_____

_____

Weight: _____

Sleep Time: _____

I am Feeling:

How will I make Tommorrow Awesome:

_____

_____

"I close my eyes in order to see."
– Paul Gauguin

Date: _____ / _____ / _____

Day 80

Breakfast:
_____
_____
_____
_____

Lunch:
_____
_____
_____
_____

Dinner:
_____
_____
_____
_____

Snacks:
_____
_____
_____
_____

Cravings / Response:
_____
_____
_____
_____

Calories Consumed: _____

Calories Burned: _____

Water Intake:

Exercise/Workout/Activity:
_____
_____
_____
_____

Weight: _____

Sleep Time: _____

I am Feeling:
😀 🙂 😐 🙁

How will I make Tommorrow Awesome:
_____
_____

*"The only person you are destined to become
is the person you decide to be."
– Ralph Waldo Emerson*

Date: _____ / _____ / _____

Day 81

Breakfast:

_____

_____

_____

_____

Lunch:

_____

_____

_____

_____

Dinner:

_____

_____

_____

_____

Snacks:

_____

_____

_____

Cravings / Response:

_____

_____

_____

Calories
Consumed: _____

Calories
Burned: _____

Water Intake:

Exercise/Workout/Activity:

_____

_____

_____

_____

_____

Weight: _____   Sleep Time: _____   I am Feeling:

How will I make Tommorrow Awesome:

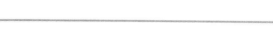

_____

"When I let go of what I am, I become what I might be."
– Lao Tzu

Date: _____ / _____ / _____

Day 82

Breakfast:
_____
_____
_____
_____

Lunch:
_____
_____
_____

Dinner:
_____
_____
_____
_____

Snacks:
_____
_____
_____

Cravings / Response:
_____
_____
_____
_____

Calories
Consumed: _____

Calories
Burned: _____

Water Intake:

Exercise/Workout/Activity:
_____
_____
_____
_____

Weight: _____   Sleep Time: _____   I am Feeling:

How will I make Tommorrow Awesome:
_____
_____

"Every moment is a fresh beginning."
– T.S. Eliot

Date: _____/ _____/ _____   Day **83**

Breakfast: Lunch: Dinner:

_____   _____   _____

_____   _____   _____

_____   _____   _____

_____   _____   _____

Snacks: Cravings / Response:

_____   _____

_____   _____

_____   _____

_____   _____

Calories   Calories   Water Intake:
Consumed: _____   Burned: _____

Exercise/Workout/Activity:

_____

_____

_____

_____

_____

Weight: _____   Sleep Time: _____   I am Feeling:

                                                        😀 🙂 😐 🙁

How will I make Tommorrow Awesome:

_____

_____

"Motivation is what gets you started.
Habit is what keeps you going."
— Jim Ryun

Date: ____/____/____

Breakfast:
_____
_____
_____
_____

Lunch:
_____
_____
_____
_____

Dinner:
_____
_____
_____
_____

Snacks:
_____
_____
_____

Cravings / Response:
_____
_____
_____

Calories Consumed: _____

Calories Burned: _____

Water Intake:

Exercise/Workout/Activity:
_____
_____
_____
_____

Weight: _____

Sleep Time: _____

I am Feeling:
😃 🙂 😐 🙁

How will I make Tommorrow Awesome:
_____
_____

*"If you ever lack the motivation to train then think
what happens to your mind & body when you don't."
– Shifu Yan Lei*

Measurements:

1. Chest: _____
2. Waist: _____
3. Hips: _____
4. Thigh: _____
5. Calf: _____
6. Arm: _____

Weekly Meal Plan:

Weekly Goals:

_____

_____

_____

How I feel about:

Diet: 😃 🙂 😐 🙁

Exercise: 😃 🙂 😐 🙁

Monday: _____
_____
_____

Tuesday: _____
_____
_____

Wednesday: _____
_____
_____

Thursday: _____
_____
_____

Friday: _____
_____
_____

Saturday: _____
_____
_____

Sunday: _____
_____
_____

Notes: _____
_____
_____

Date: ____ / ____ / _____

Day 85

Breakfast:

_____
_____
_____
_____

Lunch:

_____
_____
_____

Dinner:

_____
_____
_____
_____

Snacks:

_____
_____
_____

Cravings / Response:

_____
_____
_____
_____

Calories
Consumed: _____

Calories
Burned: _____

Water Intake:

Exercise/Workout/Activity:

_____
_____
_____
_____

Weight: _____

Sleep Time: _____

I am Feeling:

How will I make Tommorrow Awesome:

_____
_____

"You can have results or excuses, but not both."
– Arnold Schwarzenegger

Date: _____ / _____ / _____

Breakfast:

_____

_____

_____

_____

Lunch:

_____

_____

_____

_____

Dinner:

_____

_____

_____

_____

Snacks:

_____

_____

_____

Cravings / Response:

_____

_____

_____

Calories Consumed: _____

Calories Burned: _____

Water Intake:

Exercise/Workout/Activity:

_____

_____

_____

_____

Weight: _____   Sleep Time: _____

I am Feeling:

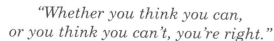

How will I make Tommorrow Awesome:

_____

_____

"Whether you think you can,
or you think you can't, you're right."
– Henry Ford

Date: _____ / _____ / _____

Breakfast: Lunch: Dinner:

_____   _____   _____

_____   _____   _____

_____   _____   _____

_____   _____   _____

Snacks: Cravings / Response:

_____   _____

_____   _____

_____   _____

_____   _____

Calories   Calories   Water Intake:
Consumed: _____   Burned: _____

Exercise/Workout/Activity:

_____

_____

_____

_____

Weight: _____   Sleep Time: _____   I am Feeling:

😃 🙂 😐 🙁

How will I make Tommorrow Awesome:

_____

_____

"The successful warrior is the average man,
with laser-like focus."
— Bruce Lee

Date: _____ / _____ / _____

Day 88

Breakfast:

_____

_____

_____

_____

Lunch:

_____

_____

_____

_____

Dinner:

_____

_____

_____

_____

Snacks:

_____

_____

_____

_____

Cravings / Response:

_____

_____

_____

_____

Calories
Consumed: _____

Calories
Burned: _____

Water Intake:

Exercise/Workout/Activity:

_____

_____

_____

_____

_____

Weight: _____

Sleep Time: _____

I am Feeling:
😃 🙂 😐 🙁

How will I make Tommorrow Awesome:

_____

_____

"You must expect great things of yourself before you can do them."
— Michael Jordan

Date: _____ / _____ / _____

Day 89

Breakfast:

_____
_____
_____
_____

Lunch:

_____
_____
_____
_____

Dinner:

_____
_____
_____

Snacks:

_____
_____
_____

Cravings / Response:

_____
_____
_____
_____

Calories Consumed: _____

Calories Burned: _____

Water Intake:

Exercise/Workout/Activity:

_____
_____
_____
_____
_____

Weight: _____

Sleep Time: _____

I am Feeling:

How will I make Tommorow Awesome:

_____
_____

"Action is the foundational key to all success."
— Pablo Picasso

Date: _____ / _____ / _____

Breakfast:

_____

_____

_____

_____

Lunch:

_____

_____

_____

_____

Dinner:

_____

_____

_____

_____

Snacks:

_____

_____

_____

Cravings / Response:

_____

_____

_____

_____

Calories
Consumed: _____

Calories
Burned: _____

Water Intake:

Exercise/Workout/Activity:

_____

_____

_____

_____

_____

Weight: _____   Sleep Time: _____   I am Feeling:

How will I make Tommorrow Awesome:

_____

_____

"Things may come to those who wait,
but only the things left by those who hustle."
– Abraham Lincoln

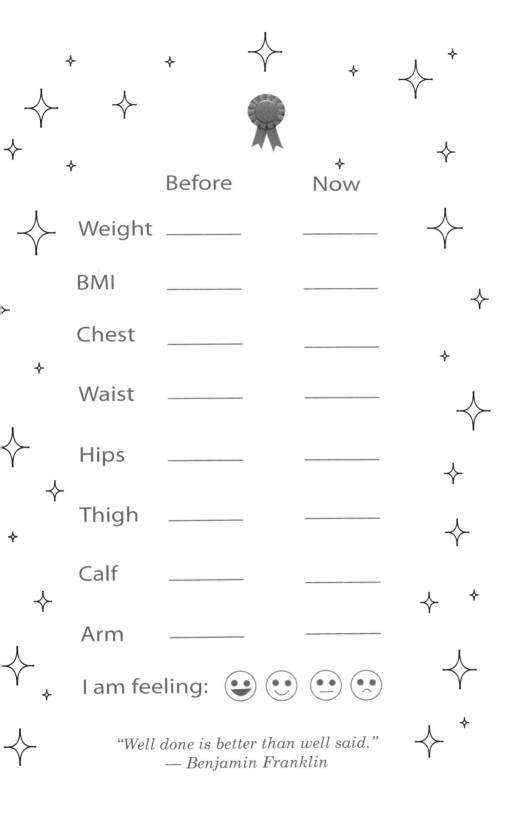

	Before	Now
Weight	_____	_____
BMI	_____	_____
Chest	_____	_____
Waist	_____	_____
Hips	_____	_____
Thigh	_____	_____
Calf	_____	_____
Arm	_____	_____

I am feeling: 😃 🙂 😐 🙁

"Well done is better than well said."
— Benjamin Franklin

Hi!

Thank you for purchasing this book.

My name is Sujatha Lalgudi. I hope you found this journal to be helpful in your diet & fitness journey.

Your kind reviews and comments will encourage me to make more books like this.

If you have any suggestions on how I can improve this book to make it more useful, please write to me at sujatha.lalgudi@gmail.com with the subject as Diet & Fitness.

I have included a coloring page in this book.

Thank you
Sujatha Lalgudi

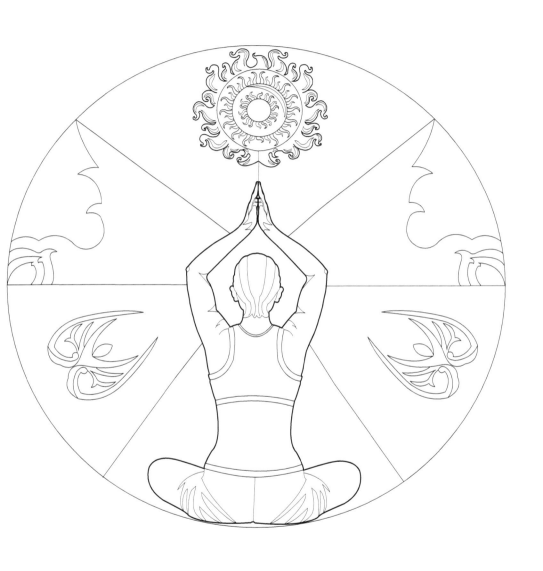

50045001R00062

Made in the USA
San Bernardino, CA
26 August 2019